I Can Be a Hero Series

The Germ Squad

Colds, Flu, and Stomach Bugs

Leeza Wilson

Printed in the United States of America.
Published by Tsarina Press

ISBN: 978-1-948429-07-8

Photos courtesy of Pixabay and by permission of Sevier County Ambulance Service and Walden's Creek Fire Department.

Legal Disclaimer

Even though I am a licensed EMT Advanced and firefighter, I am not your personal EMT. The information in this book is completely factual, however, for simplicity not all information pertaining to recognition and treatment of a diabetic emergency is relayed in this book. This book should not be used in lieu of seeking advanced medical help in an emergency. If you or a family member, friend, neighbor, or stranger in your presence is experiencing a medical emergency you should call 911.

Dedication

This series is dedicated to all the little heroes out there that have stepped up and saved a life and to the emergency workers and first responders who daily sacrifice their time, energy, and personal safety to save the lives of strangers. Special thanks to Waldens Creek Volunteer Fire Department and Sevier County Ambulance Service for your support.

Books in This Series

My Grandpa is Extra Sweet: Diabetic Emergencies

The Germ Squad: Colds, Flu, and Stomach Viruses

Where is Your Heartbeat?—Cardiac Emergencies

Preface

This book is part of a series of books that helps teach little children about different types of medical problems and emergencies and what they can do to help their friend or loved one. As an EMT and firefighter, I know how serious a medical emergency can be and how much time matters.

This series of books is designed to help children and their parents or guardians recognize the signs and symptoms of a medical emergency, know when it is appropriate to call 911, and what to do to help someone who is sick or injured while more advanced medical aid is on the way. This series of books is not intended to take the place of more advanced medical aid.

Never underestimate the ability of a young child to understand the medical conditions of family members and close friends and their ability to save a life. Many a child, including my son, have proven their ability to be little life savers and heroes.

Go over this book carefully with your child. Take the time to answer any questions they may have. If someone in your family suffers from a medical condition, such as heart trouble, and you feel your child is old enough and mature enough to understand, explain to your child the purpose of any needed medical equipment and when appropriate, how to work it if an emergency should arise in your absence. And please do not forget to explain to your child that medical equipment is not a toy and should never be played with.

The Germ Squad

Colds, Flu, and Stomach Bugs

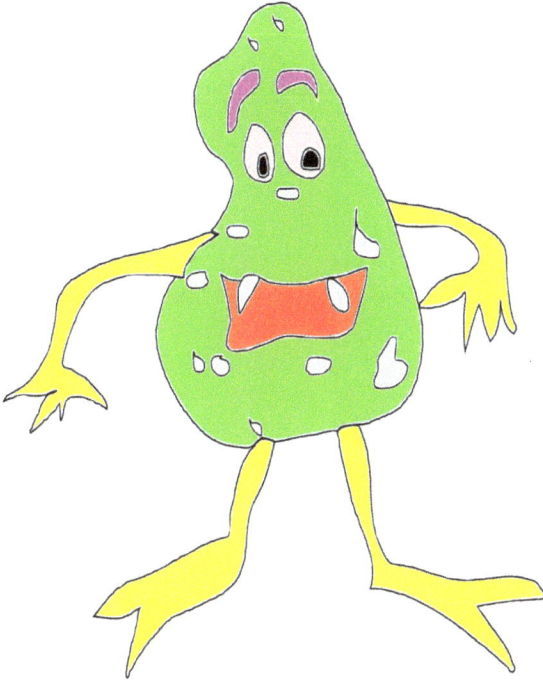

Howdy! I'm Germaine the germ, leader of the Germ
Squad. I'm an **influenza germ**. I cause the flu virus.

My friends from the Germ Squad, Ryan the **rhinovirus germ** and Nora the **norovirus germ**, and I are going to tell you all about germs and how to stay healthy.

Ryan the **rhinovirus germ** causes cold symptoms and Nora the **norovirus germ** causes the stomach flu.

We germs can be quite **contagious**, and some of us can survive for up to several weeks or months outside of the human body. We can be found in the air and on the surface of many common items that you use daily.

Let us tell you how we get there and what you can do to prevent getting sick by us and spreading us around.

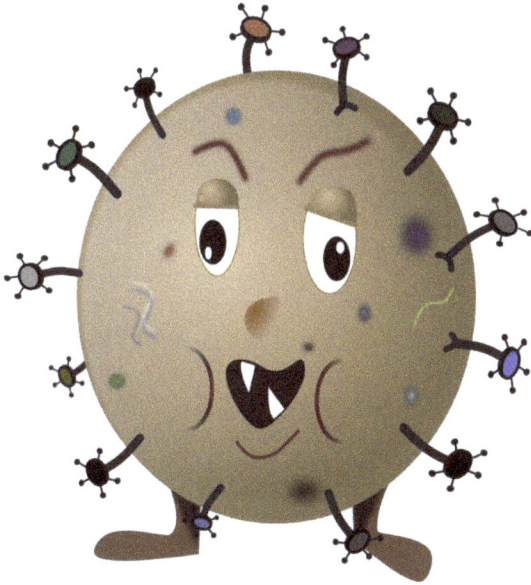

My name is Ryan the **rhinovirus germ.** I get into the air when you cough or sneeze and don't cover your mouth. We are also found on used tissues and can live on them from fifteen to forty-five minutes.

So when you blow your nose into a tissue and lay it on a table or counter, my germ friends and I can travel onto that surface from the tissue.

We get on hard and soft surfaces as we float through the air and when you touch something or someone while carrying live germs on your hands.

That means when you blow your nose, or cough or sneeze into your hand, and then touch something or someone before you wash your hands, you can transfer our germs to anything or anyone you touch.

Rhinovirus and **influenza germs** can survive on your hands up to one hour. Once we germs get on a hard surface, like a desktop or doorknob, we can survive up to twenty-four hours.

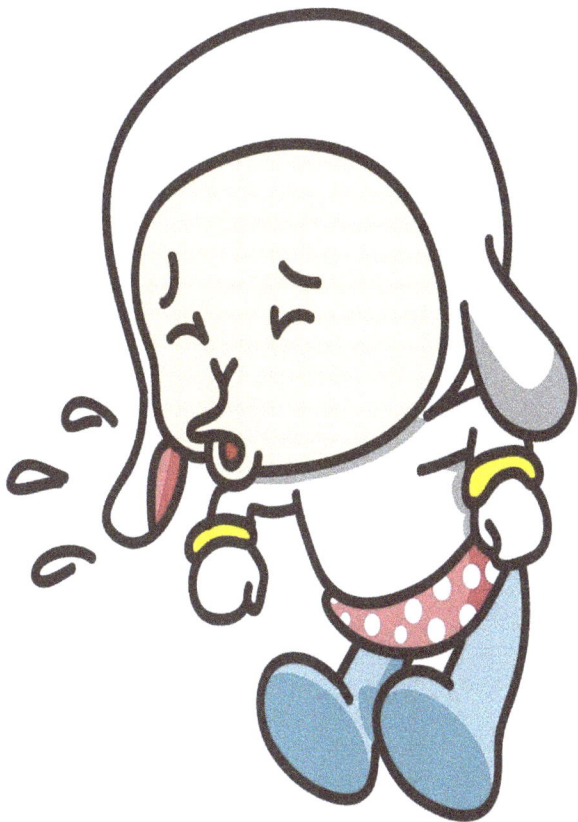

Rhinovirus germs cause cold symptoms which can include a stuffy or runny nose; a sore throat; chest congestion and cough; mild fever; tiredness; itchy, watery eyes; sneezing; headache and muscle aches.

Symptoms are usually mild, but in some people symptoms can be worse, such as high fever and severe head and or chest congestion.

If you get sick with a cold, bed rest and plenty of fluids along with a mild fever and pain reducer, and cough medicine if needed, will help you feel better in a few days.

If your symptoms are severe or lasts more than a few days, or if you begin getting worse instead of better, you should go to see your family doctor.

Unless you are experiencing life threatening symptoms, such as not being able to breathe, or altered mental status that makes you unable to stay awake or unaware of where or who you are, then you should *not* call 911. You should make an appointment with your doctor and go by personal car.

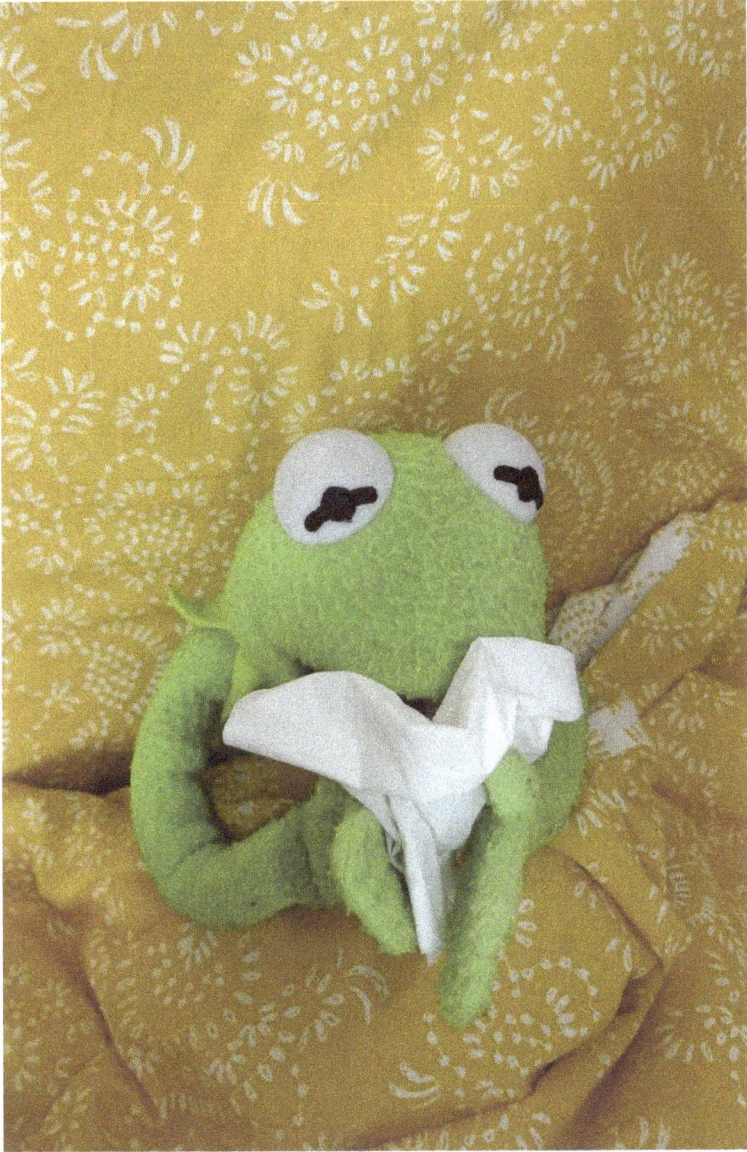

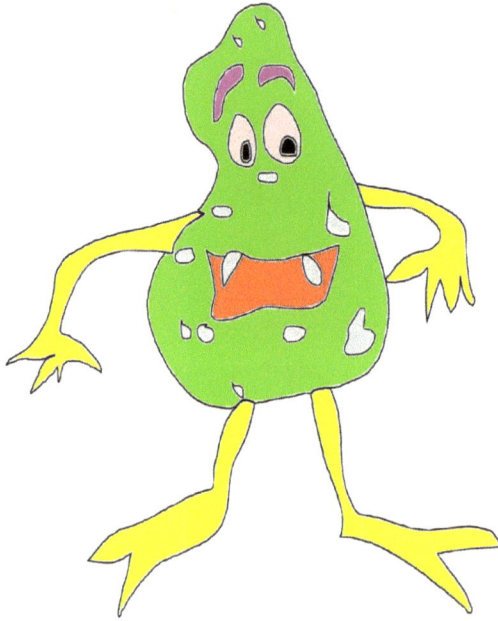

Influenza germs, like myself, are spread the same way as **rhinovirus germs**. But influenza germs cause the flu.

The flu is more severe than a cold, even though a lot of the symptoms are the same. But unlike colds, flu can cause a very high fever and severe respiratory problems.

Sometimes people get so sick because of the flu that they die. That's why it's very important to wash your hands often, avoid being around people who are sick with the flu, and go to see your doctor when you first notice symptoms of getting sick.

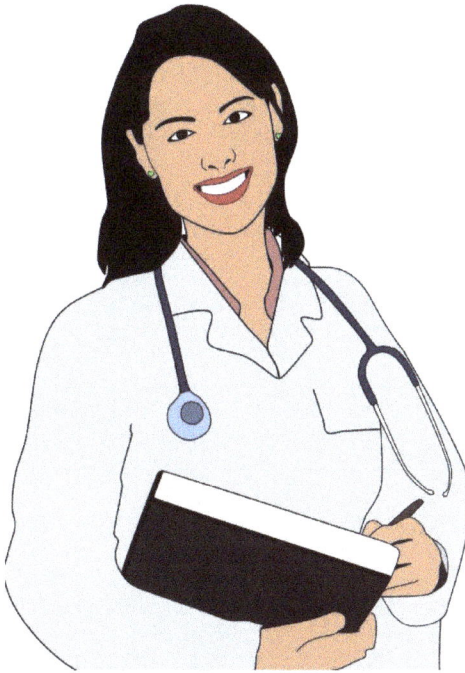

The flu can be mild to severe. Infants, small children, the elderly, and people with a suppressed immune system are at high risk for developing a severe case of the flu. These groups should always get a flu shot if they are not allergic to it.

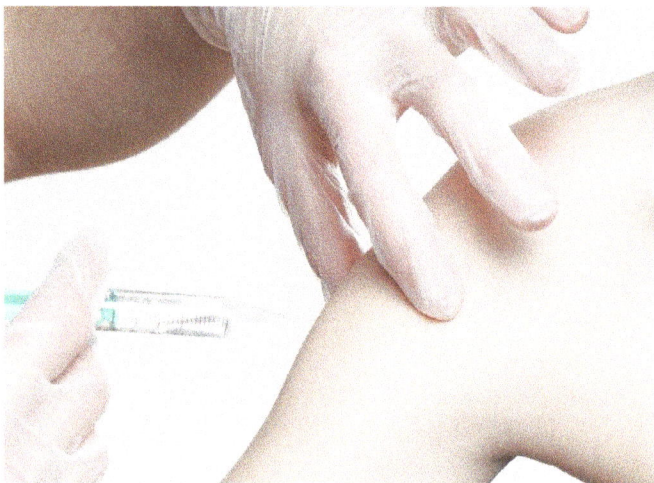

Severe cases of the flu can cause a very high fever that lasts for several days and respiratory problems that could prevent the sick person from getting enough oxygen. High fevers can also cause dehydration.

If the sick person is acting very confused, having a seizure, having severe trouble breathing, or you cannot wake them up, then you should call **911**.

To prevent catching and spreading the **rhinovirus and influenza germs** you should wash your hands after coughing or sneezing into them and after blowing your nose.

You can also prevent the spread of these germs from getting on your hands by coughing or sneezing into your sleeve near your elbow or into the top of your shirt or into a tissue.

Always throw your used tissues in a trash can and wash your hands after you blow your nose. You should wash your hands often with soap and water for at least twenty seconds, working the soap into a rich lather that covers all surfaces of your hands, fingers, and under your nails.

If you are unable to wash your hands, you may use an alcohol based hand sanitizer to help prevent the spread of germs.

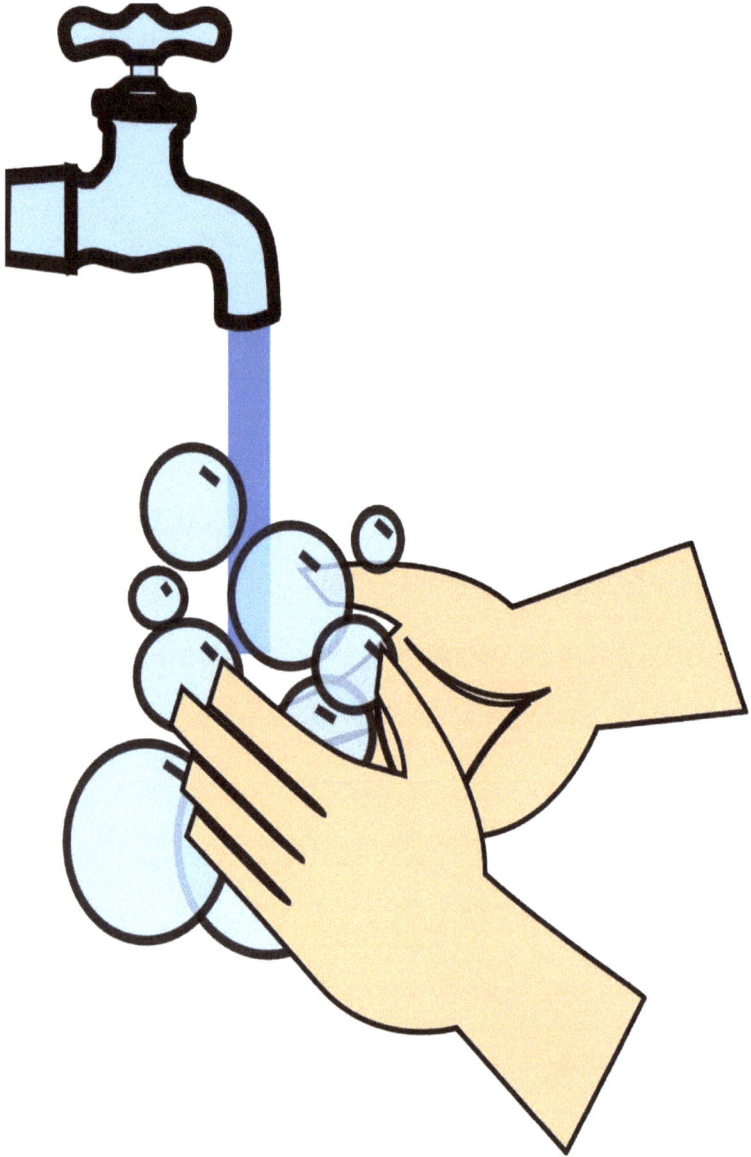

You can also prevent getting sick by always getting at least eight hours of sleep a night, eating healthy foods like fruits and vegetables, and exercising regularly. Doing these things boost your immune system which helps fight off infections and illnesses.

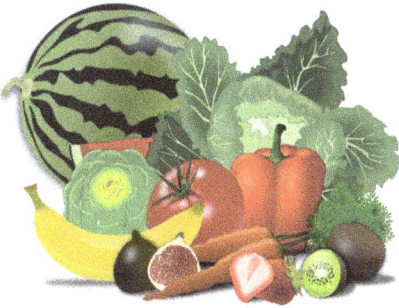

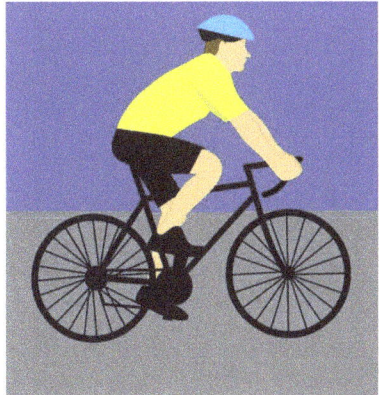

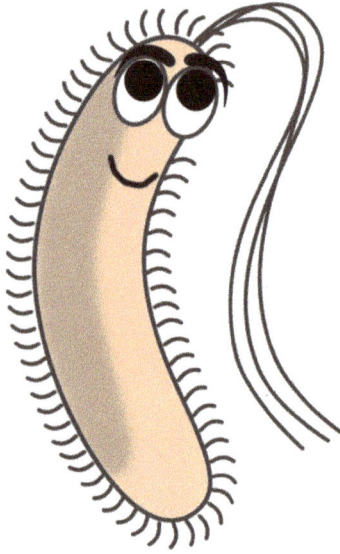

I'm Nora the **Norovirus germ**. I can make people feel pretty awful for one to three days. I cause stomach and intestinal upset.

Some people call the illness caused by germs in my family the stomach flu or stomach bug. **Norovirus** is also often the cause of **food poisoning**. Germs like me have an **incubation period** of 12-36 hours.

An **incubation period** is the time difference between when you were exposed to an illness and the first appearance of symptoms. **Norovirus germs** can survive on hard surfaces for several days or weeks.

Like my germ squad friends, Germaine and Ryan, **Norovirus germs** are spread through the air. These germs get into the air when someone sick with the virus vomits. The germs can then settle on surfaces and cause the virus to spread to others.

The virus can also be spread when someone's hands are contaminated with the virus and they touch something, like food or doorknobs.

The **Norovirus** causes nausea, mild to severe stomach cramps, vomiting, and diarrhea. Sometimes the virus also causes low-grade fever, chills, headache, and muscle aches.

If you should catch the **norovirus** or one similar to it that gives you an upset stomach, you should rest and drink lots of fluids to prevent **dehydration**.

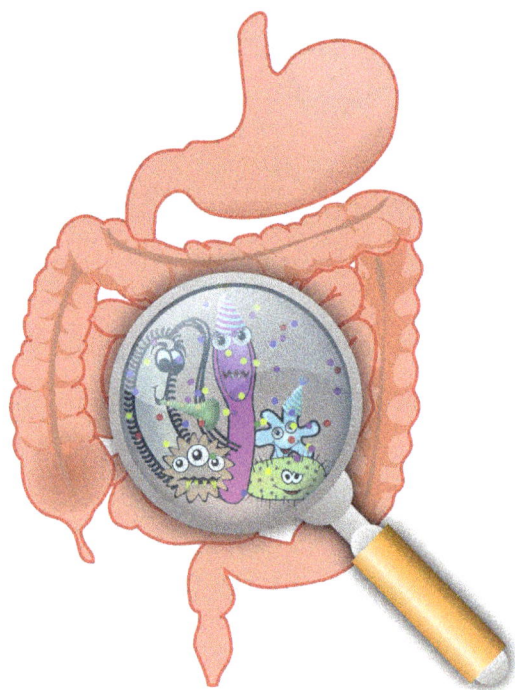

If you or someone in your family gets sick with a cold, the flu, or a stomach flu there are certain things you should do to prevent others from getting sick too.

Clean surfaces that have been exposed to germs with soap and water or a mild bleach solution. Areas that are especially important to clean are counter tops, toilets, sinks, and doorknobs.

You should always wash your hands after going to the bathroom, even if you're not sick, to prevent spreading germs to others.

Dishes and drinking glasses should be washed with warm, soapy water. Never drink behind someone else or share eating utensils because germs can be spread that way. You should also never let your mouth touch the metal spout of public drinking fountains because germs can live there even though it's a water source.

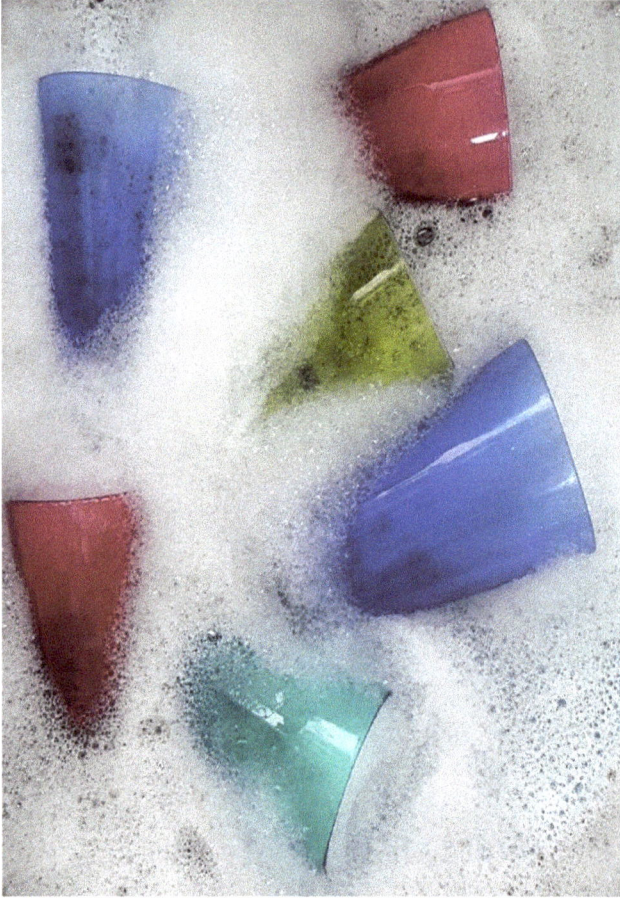

If a loved one is sick, you can be their helper and hero by bringing them something to drink or eat, making sure they are warm or cool enough, and being quiet so they can rest. You can also make sure they have tissues for their nose and a trash can close by to throw away the used ones.

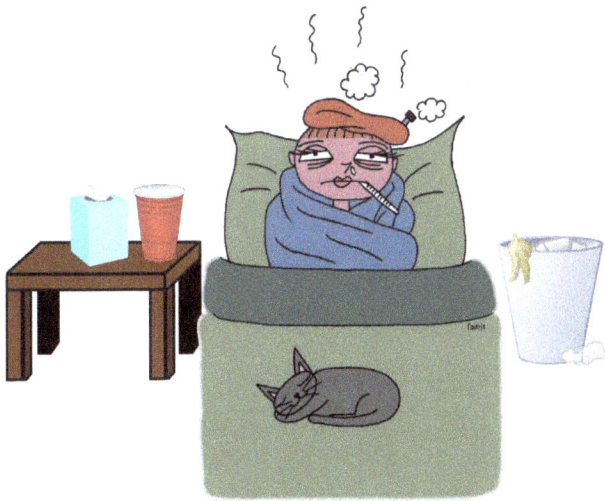

Colds and stomach bugs are rarely serious enough to cause a medical emergency. But sometimes a person can get extremely dehydrated from the stomach flu or a high fever. That can be a life-threatening situation.

A person that is severely dehydrated may not be able to pee, may have sunken eyes, a rapid heartbeat, feel dizzy, and may faint. This type of dehydration is a medical emergency and needs to be treated immediately.

If the person is unable to take liquids by mouth or keep down what they are drinking, dehydration can occur quickly. It's okay to call 911 for someone who is suffering from severe dehydration.

The paramedics and EMTs can give them saline through an IV that will help rehydrate them. If their vomiting is severe or projectile, then the paramedics can give them medicine that will calm their stomach.

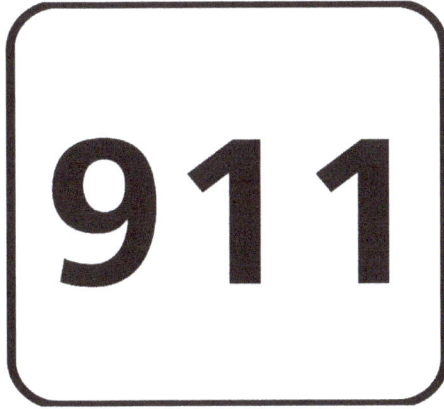

If you have to call **911,** always stay on the phone with the **911** operator until he or she tells you to hang up or until the **ambulance** or **First Responders** arrive. You will need to tell the **911** operator what your emergency is, your name, address, and possibly your phone number so they can get help to you right away.

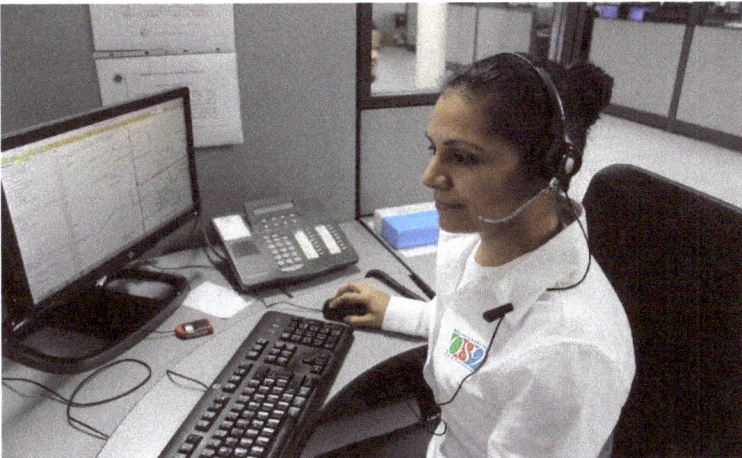

There are many more types of germs in the Germ Squad that can make you very sick. Some of these germs can cause symptoms similar to the common cold or stomach flu. And other germs can cause more serious illnesses like severe respiratory infections, Chicken pox, Measles, and strep throat. There are vaccines that prevent illnesses like Chicken pox, the flu, and Measles.

Following the safety tips in this book can protect you from germs like us and help you avoid catching an infection. Eating healthy foods, getting regular exercise, getting plenty of rest at night, and maintaining good personal hygiene will help you stay healthy and strong.

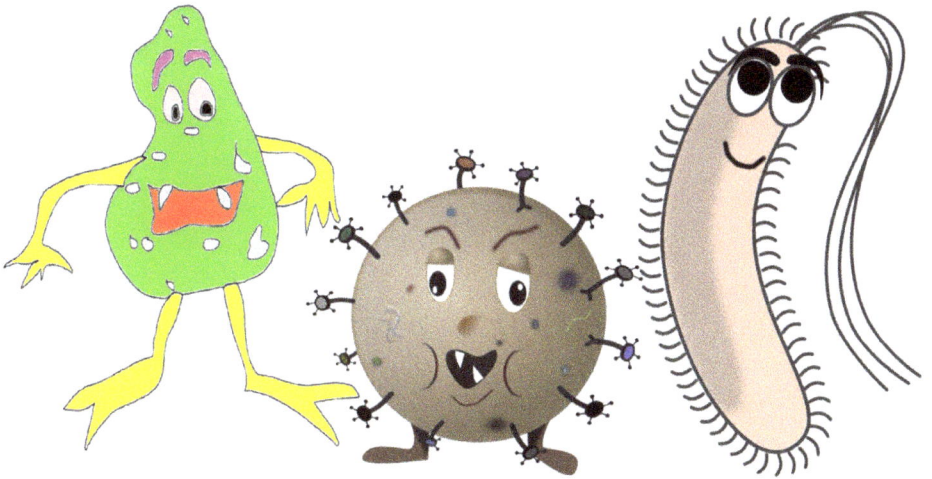

Cold/Flu Symptoms

- Congestion and/or sinus pressure

- Runny nose

- Sneezing

- Loss of smell and/or taste

- Nasal redness

- Post-nasal drip

- Body and muscle aches

- Chest congestion with or without phlegm

- Itchy, watery, red eyes

- Headache

- Swollen lymph nodes

- Sore, itchy throat

- Chills

- Fatigue

- Fever

Stomach Flu Symptoms

- Diarrhea
- Vomiting
- Nausea
- Abdominal cramping
- Mild fever
- Chills
- Headache
- Muscle aches
- Fatigue

Dehydration Symptoms
Infants and Young Children

- Dry mouth
- No tears when crying
- Sunken soft spot on top of skull, sunken eyes, and/or cheeks
- Sleepiness, lack of energy
- Dry diapers for at least 3 hours
- Irritability

Dehydration Symptoms
Adults

Mild to moderate

- Thirst
- Dry mouth
- Not peeing much
- Dark yellow pee
- Dry, cool skin
- Headache
- Muscle cramps

Severe

- Not peeing
- Very dark yellow pee
- Dizziness
- Rapid heartbeat
- Rapid breathing
- Sunken eyes
- Sleepiness, lack of energy
- Confusion or irritability
- Fainting

For Further Reading

www.medicine.net/norovirus_infection

www.medicine.net/influenza

www.medicine.net/common_cold

www.webmd.com/a-to-z-guides/dehydration-adults

Glossary

Ambulance – A vehicle that can be a van or box-shaped truck that has a cot to carry a patient on and has medical equipment to treat patients having a medical emergency. It has emergency lights and a siren to quickly respond to emergencies and get patients to a hospital quickly.

Dehydration – a condition where the body does not have a sufficient amount of water.

EMS – Emergency Medical Services. These people are trained on what to do in case of a medical emergency and can transport a person to the hospital. They can be Advanced Emergency Medical Technicians or Paramedics.

First Responders – Men and women who are medically trained in first aid and CPR who often respond with the fire department or rescue squad.

Food Poisoning – A food caused illness that may be caused by eating food that has spoiled, or contains a toxin, chemical, or infectious agent, such as a virus, bacteria, or parasite

Germs – A microorganism that causes disease or illness

Incubation period – the time between exposure to a virus or infection and the moment when symptoms first appear.

Influenza – An infectious virus that has three different strains called Type A, Type B, Type C. Symptoms can range from mild to severe.

9-1-1 – The number to call in case of an emergency to get in touch with EMS, Fire Department, or Police.

Norovirus – A variety of single-stranded RNA viruses that cause gastric illness, such as nausea, vomiting, and/or diarrhea.

Picornavirus – A group of very small single-stranded RNA viruses. Some of the viruses included in this group are rhinovirus, enterovirus, and poliovirus.

Rhinovirus –a virus that causes some forms of the common cold. It is part of the picornavirus family.

RNA – Ribonucleic acid. An acid found in all living cells. Its main purpose is to transfer messages from DNA with instructions for controlling the synthesis of proteins. Viruses of this type may be single- or double-stranded.

Saline – A salty, liquid sugar that is given through a needle in a vein.

About the Author

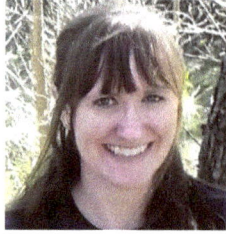

Leeza Wilson is a writer and licensed EMT Advanced in the state of Tennessee and a volunteer firefighter with Walden's Creek Volunteer Fire Department in Sevier County TN. She has always had a passion for the medical field. In 2007 she began working as an EMT with a county 911 service in South Carolina. In 2008 she began volunteering with Shepard Fire Department in Camden, South Carolina. She has a combined total of 10 years in the emergency services field.

When Leeza is not responding to emergency calls, she is writing poetry, fiction, and non-fiction for children and adults; running her publishing company; and spending time with her family.

Connect on Social Media

www.facebook.com/icanbeahero

www.twitter.com/leezatheauthor

www.instagram.com/leezatheauthor

www.facebook.com/leezatheauthor

To find out about upcoming releases in the series and other books published by Tsarina Press visit www.tsarinapress.com

Please Write a Review

Thank you for reading my book. It is my deepest wish that you had a pleasant reading experience and found this book informative and useful. Whether you did or didn't, please feel free to get in touch and let me know what you thought. I love hearing from my readers and I always try my best to respond to emails from my fans. I value your honest feedback.

As any author will tell you, reviews are so very important in helping our books get noticed. Reviews help authors reach more readers by letting them know if a book is worth reading or not. So I rely a lot on reviews to help readers find my books and know if they're worthy of investing their time in to read. It only takes a couple of minutes to write a brief review of what you thought of the book. So if you can take a minute to write an honest review, I would greatly appreciate it, even if it's a negative review. All reviews matter, whether they're 1 star or 5 stars, a small essay or just one word. Reviews can be left on Goodreads or any digital store where the book is available for sale.

Thanks!

Leeza Wilson

.

www.ingramcontent.com/pod-product-compliance
Lightning Source LLC
Chambersburg PA
CBHW051249020426
42333CB00025B/3134